Mastering Type 2 Diabetes

A Comprehensive Guide to Management and Wellness

Publish by kay Mae

Table of Contents:

Chapter 1: Introduction: Understanding Type 2 Diabetes

Type 2 diabetes is a chronic condition that affects how your body processes blood sugar (glucose). Glucose is a critical energy source for your cells, but in diabetes, either your body resists the effects of insulin—the hormone that regulates glucose—or it doesn't produce enough insulin to maintain normal glucose levels. This leads to hyperglycemia, a condition characterized by elevated blood sugar levels.

Over the past few decades, the prevalence of type 2 diabetes has risen dramatically, making it a global public health concern. According to the World Health Organization (WHO), over 400 million people worldwide are living with diabetes, and type 2 accounts for the majority of these cases.

Personal Impact and Stories

To better understand the human side of this condition, consider the story of John, a 52-year-old accountant who was diagnosed with type 2 diabetes after years of ignoring symptoms like fatigue and excessive thirst. For John, the diagnosis was a wake-up call that led to major lifestyle changes, including improved eating habits and regular exercise. Stories like John's highlight the transformative journey many face when learning to live with diabetes.

Why Understanding Diabetes Matters

Living with diabetes requires more than just managing blood sugar levels—it involves a holistic approach to health. Without proper understanding, people may face severe complications, including cardiovascular disease, kidney failure, and vision loss. Moreover, the emotional toll of managing a chronic condition can lead to stress and depression if left unaddressed.

The Economic and Social Context

Type 2 diabetes also carries a significant economic burden. In the United States alone, diabetes care costs exceed $300 billion annually. Beyond financial implications, the stigma surrounding the condition often isolates individuals, making community support crucial for mental well-being.

What This Book Offers

This book is designed to empower readers with actionable insights into managing and thriving despite a type 2 diabetes diagnosis. Each chapter delves into different aspects of the condition, from understanding its biological mechanisms to mastering lifestyle changes. By integrating expert advice, scientific research, and real-world stories, this guide aims to provide a roadmap for healthier living and greater confidence in diabetes management.

Chapter 2: The Science Behind Type 2 Diabetes

Type 2 diabetes develops gradually over time, often starting with insulin resistance. This chapter explores the physiological mechanisms behind the condition, as well as the genetic and environmental factors that contribute to its development.

Insulin and Glucose Metabolism

Insulin is a hormone produced by the pancreas that helps regulate blood sugar levels. When you eat, your body breaks down carbohydrates into glucose, which enters your bloodstream. Insulin facilitates the absorption of glucose into your cells, providing energy. In type 2 diabetes, the cells become resistant to insulin, and the pancreas struggles to produce enough to overcome this resistance. Over time, this leads to elevated blood sugar levels.

Risk Factors: Genetics and Lifestyle

Genetic Influences

Type 2 diabetes often runs in families, suggesting a strong genetic component. Researchers have identified multiple genes associated with insulin production and glucose metabolism. For instance, variations in the TCF7L2 gene are linked to a higher risk of developing the condition. Studies show that having a parent or sibling with type 2 diabetes doubles your risk, highlighting the importance of understanding family medical history.

Environmental and Lifestyle Factors

While genetics play a role, lifestyle and environmental factors
are equally influential. Obesity is a major risk factor,
particularly when excess fat is stored around the abdomen.
This type of fat can increase insulin resistance and
inflammation in the body. Sedentary behavior further
compounds the issue, as physical inactivity reduces your
body's ability to utilize glucose efficiently.

Diet also plays a significant role. High consumption of sugary
beverages and processed foods contributes to weight gain and
blood sugar spikes. On the other hand, a diet rich in whole
foods, fiber, and healthy fats can mitigate these risks.

Early Warning Signs

Prediabetes

Before type 2 diabetes develops, many individuals experience
prediabetes, a condition where blood sugar levels are elevated
but not high enough to be classified as diabetes. According to
the Centers for Disease Control and Prevention (CDC), about
96 million American adults have prediabetes, yet more than 80%
are unaware of it. Recognizing early signs, such as increased
thirst, frequent urination, and unexplained weight loss, can
prompt timely intervention to prevent progression.

Preventive Measures

Lifestyle modifications are critical for those at risk. Studies demonstrate that losing just 5-7% of body weight can reduce the likelihood of developing type 2 diabetes by up to 58%. Incorporating at least 150 minutes of moderate-intensity exercise per week, such as brisk walking, can also significantly improve insulin sensitivity.

A Closer Look: Real-World Context

Consider Mark, a 40-year-old IT professional with a sedentary lifestyle. Despite a family history of diabetes, he ignored his physician's warnings about prediabetes. After experiencing fatigue and blurred vision, he was diagnosed with type 2 diabetes. Mark's story underscores the need for awareness and early action. By adopting a healthier diet and regular exercise routine, he successfully lowered his blood sugar levels and reduced his reliance on medication.

The Bigger Picture

Understanding the science behind type 2 diabetes empowers individuals to make informed decisions about their health. By addressing both genetic predispositions and modifiable risk factors, it's possible to delay or even prevent the onset of this chronic condition. In the next chapter, we'll dive deeper into the role of diet and nutrition in blood sugar control, providing practical strategies for everyday life.

Chapter 3: Diet and Nutrition for Blood Sugar Control

What you eat plays a pivotal role in managing type 2 diabetes. This chapter will cover:

1. The Importance of Carbohydrate Counting: How to balance carbs and monitor their impact on blood sugar.

2. The Role of Fiber: Foods that slow glucose absorption and improve insulin sensitivity.

3. Meal Planning Tips: Strategies for creating diabetes-friendly meals.

Sample Meal Plan

To make these strategies actionable, here's a sample one-day meal plan tailored for blood sugar control:

- Breakfast: A bowl of oatmeal topped with fresh berries, a tablespoon of flaxseeds, and a handful of walnuts. Pair with unsweetened almond milk or water.

- Mid-Morning Snack: One hard-boiled egg and a small apple.

- Lunch: Grilled chicken salad with mixed greens, cherry tomatoes, cucumber, and a vinaigrette made with olive oil and lemon juice. Add a slice of whole-grain bread.

- Afternoon Snack: A handful of almonds and a cup of unsweetened green tea.

- **Dinner**: Baked salmon served with steamed broccoli and quinoa. Add a small side of roasted sweet potatoes.

- **Evening Snack (Optional)**: Greek yogurt (unsweetened) with a sprinkle of chia seeds.

Specific Food Recommendations

- **High-Fiber Foods**: Incorporate vegetables like spinach, broccoli, and kale. Opt for whole grains like quinoa, brown rice, and whole-grain bread.

- **Healthy Fats**: Use olive oil, avocados, nuts, and seeds to support satiety and stabilize blood sugar levels.

- **Protein Sources**: Lean meats, eggs, tofu, and legumes can help reduce post-meal glucose spikes.

- **Low-Glycemic Fruits**: Berries, cherries, and green apples are better options for managing blood sugar.

By integrating these dietary tips and meal plans into daily life, readers can create a sustainable and effective approach to blood sugar control. This practical guidance sets the stage for lasting changes and improved health outcomes.

Chapter 4: Exercise and Physical Activity for Diabetes Management

Diabetes is a chronic condition that affects millions of people worldwide, and managing it effectively requires a multi-faceted approach. Among the key elements of diabetes management, exercise and physical activity play a crucial role. Regular physical activity can help manage blood sugar levels, improve overall health, and reduce the risk of complications associated with diabetes. This article will explore the relationship between exercise and diabetes management, the benefits of physical activity for individuals with diabetes, and the types of exercises that are most effective.

The Role of Exercise in Diabetes Management

Exercise helps manage diabetes by improving insulin sensitivity and reducing blood glucose levels. Insulin is a hormone that helps the body use glucose for energy. In people with diabetes, the body either does not produce enough insulin (type 1 diabetes) or does not use insulin effectively (type 2 diabetes). This results in elevated blood glucose levels, which, if not controlled, can lead to complications such as cardiovascular disease, nerve damage, kidney damage, and vision problems.

Regular exercise has a direct impact on glucose metabolism. It helps the body use glucose more efficiently, which can reduce the amount of insulin required to control blood sugar. Exercise can also stimulate the muscles to take up glucose from the bloodstream, lowering blood sugar levels. This effect can last for hours after physical activity, which is particularly beneficial for individuals who struggle with high blood sugar levels throughout the day.

Benefits of Exercise for Diabetes Management

1. **Improved Blood Sugar Control**: One of the most significant benefits of exercise for people with diabetes is improved blood sugar control. Physical activity increases insulin sensitivity, meaning the body requires less insulin to process glucose. This can result in lower blood glucose levels, making it easier to manage diabetes.

2. **Weight Management**: Maintaining a healthy weight is critical for people with type 2 diabetes, as excess weight can contribute to insulin resistance. Exercise, particularly aerobic and strength training activities, helps burn calories and reduce fat, which can lead to weight loss. Even a modest weight loss (5-10% of body weight) can have a significant impact on blood sugar levels and overall diabetes management.

3. **Enhanced Cardiovascular Health**: Diabetes increases the risk of cardiovascular disease, including heart attacks, strokes, and peripheral artery disease. Regular physical activity strengthens the heart and improves circulation, which can

help prevent these complications. Aerobic exercises like walking, cycling, and swimming are particularly beneficial for cardiovascular health.

4. **Improved Mental Health**: Diabetes management can be stressful, and individuals with diabetes are at a higher risk of developing mental health issues such as depression and anxiety. Exercise has been shown to reduce stress, improve mood, and boost mental well-being. Physical activity stimulates the release of endorphins, which are natural mood boosters, and can help individuals with diabetes cope with the emotional challenges of living with a chronic condition.

5. **Reduced Risk of Complications**: Regular exercise helps reduce the risk of developing complications associated with diabetes. It can help prevent nerve damage (neuropathy), kidney disease (nephropathy), and retinopathy (damage to the eyes). Exercise also helps lower blood pressure and cholesterol levels, further reducing the risk of cardiovascular complications.

6. **Improved Sleep**: People with diabetes often experience sleep disturbances, which can worsen blood sugar control. Regular physical activity can improve sleep quality, which in turn can help regulate blood glucose levels. Exercise, especially aerobic activities, helps reduce symptoms of insomnia and improves overall sleep patterns.

Types of Exercises for Diabetes Management

The most effective exercise programs for diabetes management combine different types of physical activity. Each type of exercise provides unique benefits, and incorporating a variety of exercises into a weekly routine can help improve overall health and glucose control.

1. **Aerobic Exercise**: Aerobic exercises, also known as cardio, increase the heart rate and improve cardiovascular health. These exercises include activities such as walking, jogging, cycling, swimming, and dancing. Aerobic exercise is particularly effective in improving blood sugar control and promoting weight loss. For people with diabetes, the American Diabetes Association (ADA) recommends at least 150 minutes of moderate-intensity aerobic exercise per week, spread out over at least three days per week.

2. **Strength Training**: Strength training, or resistance exercise, involves working the muscles against resistance, such as lifting weights or using resistance bands. Strength training helps build lean muscle mass, which in turn improves insulin sensitivity and helps regulate blood sugar levels. The ADA recommends strength training at least two to three times per week. In addition to improving blood sugar control, strength training can increase metabolism and promote weight loss by burning fat.

3. **Flexibility and Balance Exercises**: Flexibility and balance exercises, such as yoga and Pilates, can help improve joint mobility, reduce stress, and enhance overall physical

function. These exercises are especially important for individuals with diabetes who may experience complications such as joint stiffness or neuropathy. Flexibility and balance exercises can also improve posture and help prevent falls, particularly in older adults with diabetes.

4. **High-Intensity Interval Training (HIIT)**: HIIT involves short bursts of intense exercise followed by periods of rest or low-intensity exercise. Research has shown that HIIT can be particularly effective in improving insulin sensitivity and reducing blood sugar levels. It also provides the benefits of both aerobic and strength training in a shorter period of time, making it an efficient workout for busy individuals. However, people with diabetes should consult with a healthcare provider before starting a HIIT program, especially if they have any heart conditions or other medical concerns.

Important Considerations for People with Diabetes

While exercise is beneficial for diabetes management, it is important to take certain precautions to ensure safety and maximize the benefits:

1. **Monitor Blood Sugar Levels**: It is essential for people with diabetes to monitor their blood sugar levels before, during, and after exercise. Exercise can cause blood sugar levels to drop, especially if the individual is taking insulin or medications that increase insulin production. To prevent hypoglycemia (low blood sugar), individuals should carry a

fast-acting source of glucose, such as glucose tablets or fruit juice, during exercise.

2. **Adjust Medications**: People with diabetes who are taking insulin or other blood sugar-lowering medications may need to adjust their dosages before or after exercise. It is essential to work with a healthcare provider to develop a personalized exercise plan that takes medication schedules into account.

3. **Stay Hydrated**: Exercise can lead to fluid loss through sweat, so staying hydrated is essential. People with diabetes, particularly those with kidney complications, should be mindful of fluid intake and consult their healthcare provider about how much water to drink during exercise.

4. **Wear Proper Footwear**: Individuals with diabetes, particularly those with neuropathy, are at risk of foot injuries. It is important to wear comfortable, well-fitting shoes to prevent blisters or sores. Regular foot checks are also essential to ensure that there are no injuries that could lead to infections.

5. **Start Slowly and Progress Gradually**: For individuals who are new to exercise or have been inactive, it is important to start slowly and gradually increase the intensity and duration of workouts. Starting with low-impact activities like walking or swimming can help build fitness without placing undue stress on the body.

Conclusion

Exercise and physical activity are integral components of diabetes management. Regular physical activity can improve blood sugar control, promote weight loss, reduce the risk of complications, and improve mental health. A balanced exercise routine that includes aerobic exercise, strength training, and flexibility exercises is ideal for individuals with diabetes. However, it is essential to monitor blood sugar levels, adjust medications as needed, and consult with a healthcare provider before starting a new exercise program. With the right approach, exercise can be a powerful tool in managing diabetes and improving overall health.

Chapter 5: Medications and Treatments: What You Need to Know

Type 2 diabetes (T2D) is a chronic condition in which the body either becomes resistant to the effects of insulin or doesn't produce enough insulin to maintain normal blood glucose levels. Unlike type 1 diabetes, where the body produces little to no insulin, type 2 diabetes is primarily related to insulin resistance and impaired insulin secretion. As the disease progresses, individuals may require medications in addition to lifestyle changes, such as diet and exercise, to manage their blood glucose levels effectively.

In this article, we will explore the medications and treatments available for managing type 2 diabetes, including their mechanisms of action, benefits, potential side effects, and the role of lifestyle changes in diabetes management.

The Importance of Managing Type 2 Diabetes

Effective management of type 2 diabetes is crucial to prevent long-term complications, which can include heart disease, kidney disease, nerve damage (neuropathy), vision loss (retinopathy), and poor wound healing. The primary goal of diabetes treatment is to maintain blood sugar levels within a healthy range, ideally between 70-130 mg/dL before meals and less than 180 mg/dL after meals.

In the early stages of type 2 diabetes, lifestyle interventions such as changes in diet, exercise, and weight management may be sufficient to keep blood glucose levels under control. However, over time, as insulin resistance worsens, medications may be required to help regulate blood glucose levels. Medications and treatments can work in various ways, including improving insulin sensitivity, increasing insulin secretion, or reducing glucose production in the liver.

Medications for Type 2 Diabetes

Several classes of medications are available to treat type 2 diabetes, each with its own mechanisms of action, benefits, and potential side effects. The choice of medication depends on the individual's health status, the severity of the condition, and the presence of other medical issues.

1. **Metformin**: The First-Line Treatment

Metformin is typically the first medication prescribed for type 2 diabetes. It is an oral medication that helps lower blood sugar by decreasing glucose production in the liver and improving the body's sensitivity to insulin.

- **Mechanism of Action**: Metformin works primarily by inhibiting the liver's ability to produce glucose, which reduces the amount of glucose released into the bloodstream. It also enhances insulin sensitivity, helping the body use insulin more effectively.

- **Benefits**: Metformin has been shown to effectively lower A1C (a measure of average blood glucose over three months) by about 1-2%. It is well-tolerated by most patients and is associated with a lower risk of weight gain and hypoglycemia (low blood sugar).

- **Side Effects**: The most common side effects of metformin are gastrointestinal, including nausea, diarrhea, and bloating. These side effects are often temporary and may subside over time. In rare cases, metformin can lead to a serious condition called lactic acidosis, which is a build-up of lactic acid in the bloodstream. This condition is more likely to occur in people with kidney problems, so kidney function should be monitored regularly.

2. **Sulfonylureas**: Stimulating Insulin Release

Sulfonylureas are a class of medications that help lower blood sugar by stimulating the pancreas to release more insulin.

- **Mechanism of Action**: Sulfonylureas bind to receptors on pancreatic beta cells, which stimulates the release of insulin. This increases insulin availability to help lower blood glucose levels.

- **Examples**: Common sulfonylureas include glipizide, glyburide, and glimepiride.

- **Benefits**: Sulfonylureas are generally effective in lowering blood glucose levels and can be used in combination with other medications, including metformin.

- **Side Effects**: One of the most significant risks of sulfonylureas is hypoglycemia, as they increase insulin secretion, potentially causing blood glucose to drop too low. They may also lead to weight gain, which can be problematic for people with type 2 diabetes, as excess weight contributes to insulin resistance.

3. **Thiazolidinediones (TZDs)**: Improving Insulin Sensitivity

Thiazolidinediones, also known as "glitazones," are oral medications that improve insulin sensitivity and help lower blood sugar.

- **Mechanism of Action**: TZDs work by binding to peroxisome proliferator-activated receptors (PPARs) in muscle and fat cells, increasing the body's sensitivity to insulin. This allows the body to use insulin more effectively, reducing blood sugar levels.

- **Examples**: The most common TZDs are pioglitazone and rosiglitazone.

- **Benefits**: TZDs can lower blood sugar and improve A1C levels. They also offer cardiovascular benefits, particularly pioglitazone, which has been shown to improve lipid profiles and reduce the risk of heart disease.

- **Side Effects**: TZDs are associated with weight gain and fluid retention, which can increase the risk of heart failure and edema (swelling). These medications should be used cautiously in individuals with heart disease or a history of heart failure. Additionally, TZDs may increase the risk of fractures, particularly in postmenopausal women.

4. **DPP-4 Inhibitors**: Enhancing Insulin Secretion

Dipeptidyl peptidase-4 (DPP-4) inhibitors are a class of medications that work by enhancing the body's natural insulin secretion.

- **Mechanism of Action**: DPP-4 inhibitors work by blocking the enzyme DPP-4, which breaks down incretin hormones. Incretins are hormones that stimulate insulin release in response to meals. By inhibiting DPP-4, these medications help increase insulin secretion and decrease glucose production by the liver.

- **Examples**: Sitagliptin (Januvia), saxagliptin (Onglyza), and linagliptin (Tradjenta) are common DPP-4 inhibitors.

- **Benefits**: DPP-4 inhibitors can help lower blood sugar levels without causing hypoglycemia. They are also weight-neutral, which makes them an attractive option for people with type 2 diabetes who are concerned about weight gain.

- **Side Effects**: The side effects of DPP-4 inhibitors are generally mild but may include headache, upper respiratory tract infections, and gastrointestinal issues. Rarely, these

medications can cause joint pain or pancreatitis (inflammation
of the pancreas).

5. **SGLT2 Inhibitors**: Reducing Glucose
Reabsorption

Sodium-glucose co-transporter 2 (SGLT2) inhibitors are a
class of medications that work by reducing glucose
reabsorption in the kidneys, promoting its excretion in urine.

- **Mechanism of Action**: SGLT2 inhibitors block the
SGLT2 protein in the kidneys, which is responsible for
reabsorbing glucose back into the bloodstream. By inhibiting
this protein, these medications increase glucose excretion in
urine, thereby lowering blood sugar levels.

- **Examples**: Canagliflozin (Invokana), empagliflozin
(Jardiance), and dapagliflozin (Farxiga) are common SGLT2
inhibitors.

- **Benefits**: SGLT2 inhibitors are effective at lowering
blood glucose and have been shown to provide additional
benefits, such as weight loss, lower blood pressure, and
improved cardiovascular outcomes. They may reduce the risk
of heart failure and kidney disease, making them beneficial for
people with cardiovascular issues.

- **Side Effects**: SGLT2 inhibitors can increase the risk of
urinary tract infections and genital infections due to increased
glucose in the urine. Dehydration and hypotension (low blood
pressure) are also potential side effects. Rarely, these
medications can cause diabetic ketoacidosis, a dangerous

condition where the body produces high levels of acids called ketones.

6. **GLP-1 Receptor Agonists**: Stimulating Insulin Release

Glucagon-like peptide-1 (GLP-1) receptor agonists are injectable medications that mimic the effects of a natural hormone that helps regulate blood sugar levels.

- **Mechanism of Action**: GLP-1 receptor agonists stimulate insulin release in response to meals, suppress glucagon (a hormone that raises blood sugar) secretion, and slow gastric emptying. This helps reduce blood sugar levels, especially after meals.

- **Examples**: Liraglutide (Victoza), semaglutide (Ozempic), and exenatide (Byetta) are common GLP-1 receptor agonists.

- **Benefits**: GLP-1 receptor agonists can lower blood glucose and A1C levels, promote weight loss, and improve cardiovascular health. They are particularly beneficial for individuals who need to lose weight as part of their diabetes management.

- **Side Effects**: Common side effects include nausea, vomiting, and diarrhea. These side effects often improve over time. Rarely, GLP-1 receptor agonists can cause pancreatitis or thyroid tumors, so individuals with a history of these conditions should use these medications cautiously.

Insulin Therapy for Type 2 Diabetes

In more advanced stages of type 2 diabetes, individuals may require insulin therapy, especially if other medications are no longer effective in controlling blood glucose. Insulin therapy can help provide the body with the insulin it needs to maintain normal blood sugar levels.

- **Types of Insulin**: Insulin therapy for type 2 diabetes includes rapid-acting, short-acting, intermediate-acting, and long-acting insulin types. Insulin is often administered through injections or insulin pumps.

- **Benefits**: Insulin therapy can help manage blood glucose effectively, particularly when other medications are not sufficient.

- **Side Effects**: The most common side effect of insulin therapy is hypoglycemia. Weight gain is also a concern, as insulin can promote fat storage.

Conclusion

Managing type 2 diabetes involves a combination of lifestyle changes and medications to keep blood glucose levels in check and prevent complications. Medications for type 2 diabetes work in various ways to improve insulin sensitivity, stimulate insulin secretion, reduce glucose production, and increase glucose excretion. Metformin is typically the first-line treatment, followed by other medications such as sulfonylureas, TZDs, DPP-4 inhibitors, SGLT2 inhibitors, and GLP-1 receptor agonists. In more advanced cases, insulin therapy may be required.

While medications are essential in managing diabetes, they should be combined with healthy lifestyle choices, including a balanced diet, regular physical activity, and weight management, to achieve the best outcomes. Working closely with a healthcare team is crucial for developing an individualized treatment plan that meets the specific needs of each person with type 2 diabetes.

Chapter 6: Monitoring and Managing Blood Sugar Levels

Type 2 diabetes is a chronic condition that affects how the body processes blood sugar (glucose). With type 2 diabetes, either the body becomes resistant to the insulin it produces, or the pancreas doesn't produce enough insulin. As a result, blood glucose levels become elevated, leading to a range of health complications over time. Effective management of blood sugar levels is essential to prevent the progression of diabetes-related complications, including heart disease, kidney damage, neuropathy, and vision problems.

Managing blood sugar in type 2 diabetes involves a combination of lifestyle interventions, medication, and regular monitoring. The goal is to keep blood glucose levels within a target range to prevent both short-term and long-term health issues. This article will explore the importance of monitoring blood sugar levels, the different methods of monitoring, and strategies for managing blood sugar in type 2 diabetes.

The Importance of Monitoring Blood Sugar Levels

Monitoring blood sugar is crucial for individuals with type 2 diabetes for several reasons:

"

1. **Preventing Complications**: Chronic high blood sugar can damage organs and systems in the body, leading to serious complications such as cardiovascular disease, nerve damage (neuropathy), kidney failure, and vision problems (retinopathy). Keeping blood glucose levels in check helps reduce the risk of these complications.

2. **Adjusting Treatment Plans**: Regular blood glucose monitoring allows individuals and healthcare providers to assess how well diabetes management strategies, such as medications and lifestyle changes, are working. If blood sugar levels are consistently outside the target range, adjustments can be made to medications, diet, or physical activity levels.

3. **Empowering Patients**: Monitoring blood sugar levels helps individuals with diabetes become more engaged in their own care. By tracking their blood glucose patterns, they can make informed decisions about their lifestyle choices, helping to better manage their condition.

4. **Avoiding Extreme Blood Sugar Levels**: Both high (hyperglycemia) and low (hypoglycemia) blood sugar levels can lead to immediate health risks. Hypoglycemia can cause dizziness, confusion, seizures, and loss of consciousness, while hyperglycemia can lead to diabetic ketoacidosis or hyperosmolar hyperglycemic state, both of which are life-threatening.

Methods of Monitoring Blood Sugar Levels

There are several ways to monitor blood glucose levels, ranging from simple at-home tests to more sophisticated continuous monitoring systems. The right method depends on an individual's specific needs, the severity of their diabetes, and the guidance of their healthcare provider.

1. **Self-Monitoring of Blood Glucose (SMBG)**

Self-monitoring of blood glucose (SMBG) is the most common method of checking blood sugar levels at home. This method involves using a glucometer, a small portable device that measures blood glucose levels from a drop of blood.

- **How It Works**: To perform SMBG, individuals use a lancet (a small needle) to prick their finger and obtain a drop of blood. This blood is then placed on a test strip, which is inserted into the glucometer. The device displays the blood glucose level, typically within a few seconds.

- **Frequency of Testing**: The frequency of testing depends on the individual's treatment plan, which may include taking medications such as insulin, oral diabetes medications, or lifestyle changes. People who use insulin may need to test their blood sugar several times a day, while those who manage their diabetes through diet and exercise may only need to check a few times a week or when symptoms arise.

- **Target Blood Sugar Levels**: The general target range for blood glucose levels is:

- **Before meals**: 70-130 mg/dL

- **1-2 hours after meals**: Less than 180 mg/dL

However, these targets may vary based on individual needs and healthcare provider recommendations.

2. **Continuous Glucose Monitoring (CGM)**

Continuous glucose monitoring (CGM) is an advanced method of tracking blood glucose levels throughout the day and night. CGMs are small devices that use a sensor inserted under the skin to measure glucose levels in the interstitial fluid (the fluid between cells). The sensor continuously tracks blood glucose levels, and the data is sent to a device (usually a smartphone or receiver).

- **How It Works**: The sensor, which is typically placed on the abdomen or arm, measures glucose levels every few minutes. The data is transmitted wirelessly to a receiver or smartphone app, allowing users to see real-time glucose trends. CGMs also provide alerts when blood glucose is too high or too low.

- **Benefits**: CGMs offer several advantages over traditional blood glucose testing:

  - **Real-Time Monitoring**: Users get continuous feedback on their blood sugar levels, making it easier to spot trends and adjust treatments or lifestyle factors accordingly.

  - **Fewer Fingersticks**: CGMs reduce the need for frequent finger pricks, making them a more convenient and less invasive option for people with diabetes.

  - **Hypoglycemia Alerts**: CGMs can alert users if their blood sugar is trending too low, allowing for timely intervention before hypoglycemia occurs.

- **Limitations**: While CGMs provide valuable data, they may be more expensive than traditional glucometers, and some users may find them uncomfortable. Additionally, CGMs measure glucose in the interstitial fluid, which can lag behind blood glucose levels by a few minutes.

3. **Hemoglobin A1C (HbA1c) Testing**

Hemoglobin A1C (HbA1c) is a blood test that measures the average blood glucose level over the past 2-3 months. It provides an overall picture of long-term blood sugar control and is an important tool for managing type 2 diabetes.

- **How It Works**: Glucose attaches to hemoglobin, a protein in red blood cells, and the amount of glucose bound to hemoglobin reflects the average blood sugar levels over time. The higher the average blood sugar, the higher the HbA1c level.

- **Target Levels**: The general target for HbA1c is less than 7%, though individual targets may vary based on factors such as age, comorbid conditions, and how well an individual can manage their blood sugar. An HbA1c level of 5.7% to 6.4% is considered prediabetes, while a level of 6.5% or higher indicates diabetes.

- **Benefits**: HbA1c testing provides a long-term view of blood sugar control, making it an essential tool for assessing the effectiveness of diabetes treatment over time. It is typically performed every 3-6 months, depending on an individual's treatment plan.

Managing Blood Sugar Levels

In addition to monitoring blood sugar levels, effective management of type 2 diabetes involves several strategies to maintain blood glucose within a healthy range. These include lifestyle modifications, medication, and addressing factors that influence blood sugar.

1. **Dietary Modifications**

Diet plays a key role in managing blood sugar levels. The focus should be on choosing nutrient-dense, low-glycemic foods that have a minimal impact on blood glucose.

- **Carbohydrate Management**: Since carbohydrates have the most significant effect on blood sugar, individuals with type 2 diabetes should focus on managing their carbohydrate intake. Complex carbohydrates (e.g., whole grains, vegetables, and legumes) are better choices than refined carbs and sugars, as they are digested more slowly and cause a more gradual rise in blood sugar.

- **Meal Planning**: Some individuals with diabetes find it helpful to work with a registered dietitian to create a meal plan that balances carbohydrates, protein, and fats. This may include portion control, eating smaller meals more frequently, and avoiding large blood sugar spikes after meals.

- **Fiber Intake**: High-fiber foods such as vegetables, fruits, legumes, and whole grains help slow the absorption of glucose and improve blood sugar control.

2. **Physical Activity**

Regular physical activity can significantly improve insulin sensitivity, reduce blood sugar levels, and aid in weight management.

- **Aerobic Exercise**: Activities like walking, cycling, swimming, and jogging can help lower blood sugar levels by increasing insulin sensitivity and encouraging the muscles to take up glucose more efficiently.

- **Strength Training**: Resistance exercises, such as weight lifting, can increase muscle mass, which helps improve insulin sensitivity and glucose uptake by the muscles.

- **Consistency**: Aim for at least 150 minutes of moderate-intensity aerobic exercise per week, along with muscle-strengthening activities on two or more days per week.

3. **Medications**

For many individuals with type 2 diabetes, lifestyle changes alone may not be sufficient to control blood sugar levels. In these cases, medications may be prescribed to help regulate blood glucose.

- **Common Medications**: Common classes of medications for type 2 diabetes include metformin (which improves insulin sensitivity), sulfonylureas (which stimulate insulin production), DPP-4 inhibitors, GLP-1 receptor agonists, SGLT2 inhibitors, and insulin therapy in advanced cases.

4. **Stress Management and Sleep**

Stress can raise blood sugar levels by triggering the release of hormones like cortisol and adrenaline. Practicing relaxation techniques such as deep breathing, meditation, and yoga can help reduce stress. Similarly, getting adequate sleep (7-9 hours per night) is essential for blood sugar control, as poor sleep can impair insulin sensitivity and increase hunger hormones.

Conclusion

Monitoring and managing blood sugar levels is a cornerstone of type 2 diabetes care. Regular blood glucose testing, whether through self-monitoring, continuous glucose monitoring, or periodic HbA1c testing, provides the data needed to make informed decisions about treatment. Effective management requires a combination of lifestyle changes, such as a balanced diet, regular physical activity, stress management, and, when necessary, medications. By staying vigilant and working closely with healthcare providers, individuals with type 2 diabetes can maintain healthy blood sugar levels and reduce the risk of complications, leading to a better quality of life.

Chapter 7: Stress Management and Mental Health in Diabetes Care

Type 2 diabetes (T2D) is a chronic condition that requires continuous attention to manage blood sugar levels, maintain overall health, and prevent complications. While much focus is placed on the physical aspects of managing diabetes—such as diet, exercise, and medication—mental health and stress management are equally critical to effective diabetes care. Stress can significantly impact blood sugar levels, and poor mental health can complicate diabetes management, leading to worse outcomes over time.

This article explores the relationship between stress, mental health, and type 2 diabetes, and offers strategies to help individuals manage stress and improve their mental well-being as part of their overall diabetes care.

The Connection Between Stress and Type 2 Diabetes

Stress, whether physical or emotional, activates the body's "fight or flight" response, triggering the release of hormones such as cortisol and adrenaline. These hormones prepare the body to deal with a perceived threat by increasing heart rate, boosting energy levels, and raising blood sugar levels. For individuals with type 2 diabetes, this response can have negative consequences, as elevated stress hormones can interfere with insulin function and increase blood glucose levels.

For example, cortisol, often referred to as the "stress hormone," raises blood sugar by prompting the liver to release stored glucose. Under normal circumstances, insulin helps regulate blood glucose levels, but in people with insulin resistance, as is common in type 2 diabetes, the body's ability to control blood sugar can be compromised. Chronic stress can thus exacerbate blood sugar instability, making it harder to maintain a healthy range of glucose levels.

Mental Health and Type 2 Diabetes

Mental health disorders, such as depression, anxiety, and diabetes distress, are common among individuals with type 2 diabetes. These conditions can have a direct impact on diabetes self-management, including diet, exercise, medication adherence, and overall motivation to maintain blood sugar control.

1. **Depression and Diabetes**

Depression is one of the most common mental health conditions in individuals with type 2 diabetes. Studies have shown that people with diabetes are at a higher risk of developing depression compared to the general population. Depression can affect many aspects of diabetes care, including self-care behaviors and treatment adherence.

- **Impact on Self-Care**: Individuals with depression may struggle with the motivation needed to follow a healthy diet, engage in regular physical activity, or take medications as prescribed. The emotional toll of diabetes, combined with the physical symptoms of depression (e.g., fatigue, lack of interest), can lead to neglect of self-care routines.

- **Blood Sugar Management**: Depression can also lead to poor blood sugar control. Elevated blood glucose levels can, in turn, worsen symptoms of depression, creating a vicious cycle. The negative emotional impact of managing a chronic condition can create a sense of helplessness and contribute to feelings of hopelessness.

2. **Anxiety and Diabetes**

Anxiety is another common mental health issue in people with type 2 diabetes. Anxiety can arise from worries about managing the disease, fear of complications, or concerns about lifestyle changes required for diabetes management.

- **Fear of Hypoglycemia**: One specific area of anxiety for people with diabetes is the fear of hypoglycemia (low blood sugar), which can occur as a result of insulin use or medication. The fear of experiencing hypoglycemia may make individuals hesitant to adjust their medications or take appropriate actions to control blood sugar levels.

- **Overworrying About Blood Sugar**: Some individuals may become excessively concerned with the fluctuations in their blood glucose levels, leading to constant checking of blood sugar or anxiety about making the wrong choices regarding diet or exercise. This can create stress and make diabetes management feel overwhelming.

3. **Diabetes Distress**

Diabetes distress is a term used to describe the emotional burden that comes with managing a chronic condition like diabetes. It is distinct from depression but can include feelings of frustration, guilt, or burnout. Diabetes distress occurs when an individual feels overwhelmed by the demands of managing the disease, which can lead to a sense of inadequacy or inability to cope.

- **Emotional Strain**: Diabetes distress can stem from the daily challenges of monitoring blood sugar levels, managing medication, and maintaining a healthy lifestyle. This emotional strain can make it harder to maintain the motivation and commitment needed for long-term diabetes management.

- **Impact on Quality of Life**: The constant attention required for diabetes care can interfere with an individual's social life, work, and relationships, leading to decreased quality of life. Feeling isolated or unsupported can exacerbate diabetes distress, which can ultimately affect physical health.

Strategies for Stress Management and Mental Health Improvement

Given the significant impact that stress and mental health can have on diabetes management, it is essential for individuals with type 2 diabetes to incorporate stress management techniques and mental health support into their care plan. Here are several strategies that can help manage stress and improve mental well-being:

1. **Mindfulness and Relaxation Techniques**

Mindfulness and relaxation techniques are powerful tools for managing stress. These practices help individuals focus on the present moment and reduce feelings of anxiety and tension.

- **Mindfulness Meditation**: Mindfulness meditation involves focusing attention on the present moment without judgment. Regular practice has been shown to reduce stress, improve emotional regulation, and enhance overall well-being. For individuals with type 2 diabetes, mindfulness meditation can help reduce the emotional impact of managing the disease and promote a more balanced approach to daily challenges.

- **Deep Breathing Exercises**: Simple deep breathing exercises can activate the body's relaxation response, lowering cortisol levels and reducing stress. Taking slow, deep breaths can also help individuals regain focus and calmness in stressful situations, such as before a medical appointment or when experiencing a blood sugar spike.

2. **Physical Activity and Exercise**

Regular physical activity is not only essential for managing blood glucose levels but also plays a significant role in reducing stress and improving mental health.

- **Exercise and Endorphins**: Physical activity stimulates the release of endorphins, which are natural mood elevators that promote feelings of well-being. Exercise can also reduce symptoms of anxiety and depression by decreasing the levels of stress hormones such as cortisol.

- **Stress Reduction Through Movement**: Activities such as walking, swimming, cycling, and yoga can help individuals with diabetes manage their weight, improve insulin sensitivity, and reduce stress levels. Incorporating exercise into daily routines can serve as both a physical and mental health tool, offering relief from the emotional challenges of managing diabetes.

3. **Social Support and Community**

Having a strong support system is crucial for managing the emotional aspects of type 2 diabetes. Social support can come from family, friends, healthcare professionals, or diabetes support groups.

- **Support Groups**: Participating in a diabetes support group can help individuals feel understood and less isolated in their experience. These groups provide a safe space for sharing challenges and successes, and they can help people develop coping strategies for managing the emotional toll of the disease.

- **Open Communication with Healthcare Providers**: Healthcare providers can be a valuable source of emotional support and guidance. Regular communication with a diabetes care team can help address concerns about managing the disease and offer strategies for coping with stress and mental health challenges.

4. **Cognitive Behavioral Therapy (CBT)**

Cognitive behavioral therapy (CBT) is a well-established form of psychotherapy that can help individuals address negative thought patterns and behaviors related to stress and mental health. CBT can be particularly beneficial for people with diabetes who experience anxiety, depression, or diabetes distress.

- **Changing Thought Patterns**: CBT helps individuals identify and challenge unhelpful thoughts and beliefs about their ability to manage diabetes. By reframing negative thinking, individuals can build a more positive outlook and improve their self-efficacy (belief in their ability to manage the condition).

- **Problem-Solving Skills**: CBT also teaches individuals effective problem-solving skills to help them cope with the day-to-day challenges of diabetes management. This can help reduce feelings of helplessness and increase confidence in their ability to manage both the physical and emotional aspects of the disease.

5. **Medication for Mental Health**

In some cases, medication may be necessary to manage mental health conditions such as depression or anxiety, which can complicate diabetes management. Antidepressant and anti-anxiety medications, when prescribed and monitored by a healthcare provider, can help improve mood and reduce feelings of emotional distress.

- **Medications for Depression and Anxiety**: Selective serotonin reuptake inhibitors (SSRIs) and other classes of antidepressants can help regulate mood and improve mental health. Anti-anxiety medications may also be prescribed for individuals experiencing high levels of anxiety related to diabetes management.

- **Integrating Mental Health with Diabetes Care**: It's important for individuals with diabetes and mental health issues to work with their healthcare providers to ensure that both physical and mental health needs are being addressed.

Mental health treatment should be considered as part of a comprehensive diabetes care plan.

Conclusion

Stress management and mental health support are integral components of effective type 2 diabetes care. Chronic stress and mental health conditions such as depression, anxiety, and diabetes distress can interfere with blood glucose management, leading to worsened health outcomes. By recognizing the impact of stress and mental health on diabetes care, individuals can take proactive steps to manage their emotional well-being. Strategies such as mindfulness, physical activity, social support, cognitive behavioral therapy, and medication can help individuals reduce stress, improve mental health, and optimize diabetes management. A holistic approach that includes both physical and mental health care is essential for achieving the best possible outcomes in type 2 diabetes.

Chapter 8: Preventing Complications: Eyes, Kidneys, and Heart Health

Type 2 diabetes is a chronic condition that can lead to a range of complications if not properly managed. Over time, high blood sugar levels can damage various organs and systems in the body, leading to severe health problems, including issues with the eyes, kidneys, and heart. These complications are some of the most common and serious concerns for individuals living with diabetes. However, with proactive management of blood glucose levels, regular monitoring, and lifestyle changes, many of these complications can be prevented or at least delayed.

In this article, we will explore the most common complications related to the eyes, kidneys, and heart in individuals with type 2 diabetes, the mechanisms behind their development, and the strategies for preventing them.

1. **Eye Health: Diabetic Retinopathy and Vision Loss**

Diabetic retinopathy is one of the leading causes of blindness in adults with type 2 diabetes. It occurs when high blood glucose levels cause damage to the small blood vessels in the retina, the light-sensitive layer at the back of the eye. As these blood vessels become weakened or blocked, it can result in vision problems, ranging from mild blurriness to complete vision loss.

How Diabetic Retinopathy Develops

Over time, uncontrolled blood sugar can lead to increased pressure in the blood vessels of the retina. This pressure damages the blood vessels, causing them to leak fluid or become blocked. In more advanced stages, new, fragile blood vessels may grow in an attempt to compensate for the damage, but these new vessels are often weak and prone to bleeding. The accumulation of blood or fluid in the retina can impair vision.

There are three stages of diabetic retinopathy:

- **Mild Nonproliferative Retinopathy (NPDR)**: Early stage where blood vessels in the retina are weakened but no significant vision impairment has occurred.

- **Moderate to Severe NPDR**: Blood vessels become more damaged, and the retina receives less oxygen, leading to swelling and further damage.

- **Proliferative Diabetic Retinopathy (PDR)**: The most advanced stage, where new blood vessels grow in the retina, causing bleeding and scarring, which can lead to vision loss.

Prevention and Management of Diabetic Retinopathy

Preventing diabetic retinopathy revolves around managing blood glucose levels, blood pressure, and cholesterol:

- **Blood Sugar Control**: Keeping blood glucose levels within a target range is crucial in preventing damage to the blood vessels in the eyes. Tight blood sugar control has been shown to reduce the risk of developing diabetic retinopathy and slow its progression.

- **Regular Eye Exams**: Early detection through regular eye exams by an eye care professional is key. Individuals with diabetes should have a dilated eye exam at least once a year to check for signs of retinopathy and other potential issues, such as cataracts and glaucoma.

- **Blood Pressure and Cholesterol Management**: Managing hypertension and high cholesterol is essential in preventing eye complications. Medications may be prescribed to control blood pressure and cholesterol, reducing the strain on the blood vessels in the eyes.

2. **Kidney Health: Diabetic Nephropathy and Kidney Disease**

Kidney disease is another significant complication of type 2 diabetes. Diabetic nephropathy, or diabetic kidney disease, occurs when the small blood vessels in the kidneys become damaged due to prolonged high blood sugar levels. The kidneys' ability to filter waste from the blood is impaired, and

over time, this damage can lead to kidney failure if left
untreated.

How Diabetic Nephropathy Develops

High blood sugar causes damage to the blood vessels in the
kidneys, which can lead to an increase in the amount of
protein (albumin) in the urine—a key indicator of kidney
damage. Early stages of kidney disease may not show
symptoms, but as the condition progresses, individuals may
experience swelling, high blood pressure, and eventually
kidney failure.

There are several stages of diabetic nephropathy:

- **Stage 1 (Normal Kidney Function)**: Early on, the
kidneys filter waste as usual, but minor damage to the blood
vessels begins to occur.

- **Stage 2 (Microalbuminuria)**: Small amounts of protein
begin to leak into the urine, a sign of early kidney damage.

- **Stage 3-4 (Macroalbuminuria)**: Larger amounts of
protein leak into the urine, and kidney function begins to
decline significantly.

- **Stage 5 (Kidney Failure)**: The kidneys no longer
function effectively, and dialysis or a kidney transplant may be
required.

**Prevention and Management of Diabetic
Nephropathy**

Preventing diabetic nephropathy involves controlling blood glucose, blood pressure, and reducing other risk factors:

- **Blood Sugar Control**: Tight control of blood glucose is the most important factor in preventing kidney damage. Keeping blood sugar levels within a healthy range reduces the strain on the kidneys.

- **Blood Pressure Control**: High blood pressure can worsen kidney damage. Medications, such as angiotensin-converting enzyme (ACE) inhibitors or angiotensin II receptor blockers (ARBs), may be prescribed to help protect the kidneys and lower blood pressure.

- **Regular Screening for Kidney Damage**: People with diabetes should have their urine checked regularly for albumin (protein) as part of routine screening. Early detection allows for timely intervention to slow the progression of kidney disease.

- **Healthy Lifestyle**: Eating a balanced diet, exercising regularly, and maintaining a healthy weight help reduce the risk of kidney disease. Avoiding smoking and excessive alcohol consumption can also protect kidney health.

3. **Heart Health: Cardiovascular Disease and Heart Attack Risk**

Cardiovascular disease (CVD) is one of the leading causes of death among individuals with type 2 diabetes. The risk of developing heart disease is significantly higher in people with diabetes due to factors such as high blood sugar, high blood

pressure, and abnormal cholesterol levels. People with
diabetes are also more likely to have atherosclerosis, where the
blood vessels become clogged with fatty deposits, restricting
blood flow to the heart and other organs.

How Diabetes Affects the Heart

Prolonged high blood sugar levels damage the blood vessels
and increase inflammation, making it easier for plaque to build
up in the arteries. This increases the risk of coronary artery
disease (CAD), which can lead to heart attacks, stroke, and
other cardiovascular complications.

There are several key factors that contribute to the increased
risk of heart disease in people with diabetes:

- **Insulin Resistance**: Insulin resistance, which is a
hallmark of type 2 diabetes, contributes to higher levels of
blood glucose and triglycerides and lower levels of HDL
(good) cholesterol. These factors increase the risk of
atherosclerosis and heart disease.

- **High Blood Pressure**: Hypertension, or high blood
pressure, is more common in individuals with diabetes and
puts additional strain on the heart and blood vessels,
increasing the risk of heart attacks and strokes.

- **Dyslipidemia**: Abnormal levels of cholesterol (e.g., high
LDL or "bad" cholesterol and low HDL cholesterol) are
often seen in people with diabetes, further contributing to
heart disease risk.

Prevention and Management of Cardiovascular Disease

Managing heart health is an essential part of preventing complications in type 2 diabetes. The following steps can help reduce the risk of cardiovascular disease:

- **Blood Sugar Control**: Tight control of blood glucose is vital for reducing the risk of heart disease. Keeping blood sugar within the target range helps prevent the damage that high blood sugar can cause to the blood vessels.

- **Blood Pressure and Cholesterol Management**: Regular monitoring of blood pressure and cholesterol levels is essential. If necessary, medications such as statins (for cholesterol) and ACE inhibitors (for blood pressure) may be prescribed to protect the heart and blood vessels.

- **Healthy Diet**: A heart-healthy diet is crucial for preventing cardiovascular disease. A diet rich in fruits, vegetables, whole grains, lean proteins, and healthy fats can help manage both blood sugar and cholesterol levels. Reducing sodium intake can also help manage blood pressure.

- **Regular Physical Activity**: Exercise is one of the most effective ways to improve heart health. Regular aerobic activity can lower blood pressure, improve cholesterol levels, and help with weight management.

- **Weight Management**: Maintaining a healthy weight is critical in reducing the risk of heart disease and managing diabetes. Losing even a small amount of weight can improve blood sugar control and reduce cardiovascular risk.

Conclusion

Diabetes-related complications affecting the eyes, kidneys, and heart can have severe consequences if not effectively managed. However, the risk of developing these complications can be significantly reduced with proper management of blood sugar levels, blood pressure, and cholesterol. Regular monitoring, lifestyle modifications, and adherence to prescribed medications are essential in preventing or slowing the progression of complications such as diabetic retinopathy, nephropathy, and cardiovascular disease.

By maintaining a comprehensive care plan that includes careful attention to eye, kidney, and heart health, individuals with type 2 diabetes can significantly improve their quality of life and reduce the risk of life-threatening complications. Regular consultations with healthcare providers and a proactive approach to diabetes management are key to ensuring long-term health and well-being.

Chapter 9: Building a Support System for Diabetes Care

Managing type 2 diabetes (T2D) requires not just medical intervention but a holistic approach that incorporates lifestyle changes, consistent monitoring, and emotional well-being. While many people with diabetes may initially focus on managing their blood sugar levels through diet, exercise, and medication, one of the most important aspects of long-term success in diabetes care is building a strong support system. Having a network of family, friends, healthcare professionals, and support groups can make the process of managing diabetes less overwhelming, provide emotional encouragement, and improve overall outcomes.

In this article, we will explore the importance of building a support system for individuals with type 2 diabetes, how to establish this system, and the roles of different members of that support network in promoting effective diabetes care.

The Importance of a Support System in Diabetes Care

Managing type 2 diabetes is a lifelong commitment that requires adherence to a complex routine of healthy eating, regular physical activity, monitoring blood glucose levels, and taking medications. The emotional, psychological, and physical demands of managing diabetes can be significant, and without support, individuals may feel overwhelmed, isolated, or discouraged. A support system offers the following benefits:

1. **Emotional Support**

Diabetes can sometimes feel like a constant battle, especially if blood glucose levels fluctuate unpredictably or if complications arise. The stress and frustration that can accompany managing a chronic condition are real and can lead to emotional exhaustion. Having emotional support from others helps reduce feelings of isolation and frustration. It provides an outlet to share struggles, receive empathy, and feel understood.

2. **Motivation and Accountability**

A strong support system plays a key role in motivating individuals with type 2 diabetes to stick to their treatment plan. Whether it's encouraging healthy eating, exercising regularly, or staying consistent with medication, having someone to check in with can help hold individuals accountable. Family, friends, or a healthcare team can encourage their loved ones to stay committed to their health goals, which is essential in managing diabetes effectively.

3. **Knowledge and Guidance**

Building a support system is not just about emotional support, but also about gaining knowledge and practical advice. Healthcare providers, diabetes educators, and nutritionists are integral members of a support system who can provide expert advice on managing the condition. Having access to accurate information and professional guidance helps individuals make informed decisions about their care.

4. **Sharing the Burden**

Managing diabetes can feel overwhelming at times, especially for those who are doing it alone. A supportive network helps share the burden of care. Whether it's helping with meal prep, accompanying someone to doctor's appointments, or providing encouragement during difficult times, sharing responsibilities can alleviate stress and improve the overall experience of living with diabetes.

5. **Improved Health Outcomes**

Studies show that individuals with a strong support system are more likely to experience better diabetes outcomes. The combination of emotional support, motivation, and practical assistance leads to better adherence to medication, improved blood sugar control, and a higher quality of life. Supportive relationships also help reduce the likelihood of developing diabetes-related complications by encouraging proactive management.

Building Your Diabetes Support System

Creating a strong, supportive network involves identifying the right people, resources, and strategies to integrate into your daily life. Below are some key components to consider when building your support system:

1. **Family and Friends**

While the healthcare team provides clinical guidance, family and friends often provide the most day-to-day support. These are the people who are closest to you and can offer both emotional and practical help. Building a support system with them begins with clear communication and mutual understanding of the challenges involved in managing diabetes.

- **Education and Awareness**: One of the first steps in involving family and friends is educating them about diabetes. Understanding what type 2 diabetes is, how it's managed, and the emotional and physical challenges it presents will help them provide better support. Encourage open conversations about your needs, whether it's help with meal planning, exercising together, or offering emotional support during challenging times.

- **Setting Boundaries and Expectations**: It's important to set realistic boundaries with family and friends. Diabetes care requires ongoing management, and loved ones should understand that their role is to support and encourage rather than take over the management of your condition. For example, if you need someone to help with grocery shopping, be specific about the types of foods you need, rather than expecting them to manage your diet completely.

- **Shared Activities**: Engage in health-focused activities together, such as going for walks, cooking healthy meals, or participating in exercise classes. This can strengthen the bond between you and your loved ones while encouraging a healthier lifestyle for everyone.

2. **Healthcare Providers**

Healthcare professionals are essential members of any diabetes support system. These professionals help with medical management, offer guidance on lifestyle changes, and provide specialized expertise that can be invaluable in managing the condition.

- **Primary Care Physician**: Your primary care doctor is the first point of contact in managing your diabetes. They are responsible for prescribing medications, monitoring your overall health, and referring you to specialists when needed. Building a strong, open relationship with your doctor is crucial for effective diabetes care.

- **Endocrinologist**: An endocrinologist is a doctor who specializes in diabetes and other hormone-related conditions. For individuals with more complex diabetes cases or those struggling to maintain blood sugar control, an endocrinologist may be necessary to provide specialized care and advice.

- **Diabetes Educator**: A certified diabetes educator (CDE) can help you understand how to monitor blood sugar, adjust medications, manage diet, and incorporate exercise into your daily life. They are an invaluable resource for education and can help you develop a personalized diabetes management plan.

- **Dietitian and Nutritionist**: Proper nutrition is a cornerstone of diabetes management. A dietitian can help you understand how to plan meals, read food labels, and make healthier food choices. Having a nutritionist who understands your specific needs can help you maintain stable blood sugar levels while enjoying food.

- **Mental Health Professionals**: Diabetes can take a toll on mental health, and seeking guidance from a therapist or counselor can be an important part of your support system. They can help you manage the emotional burden of diabetes, address feelings of anxiety or depression, and offer coping strategies for dealing with stress.

3. **Support Groups**

Support groups, whether in-person or online, offer a unique opportunity to connect with others who are going through similar experiences. These groups provide a sense of community and allow for the sharing of personal stories, tips, and encouragement.

- **Diabetes-Specific Support Groups**: Many hospitals, clinics, and diabetes organizations offer support groups for individuals with type 2 diabetes. These groups provide a safe space to discuss the challenges of managing diabetes and learn from others' experiences. They can help combat feelings of isolation and provide valuable advice from people who truly understand what you're going through.

- **Online Communities**: There are many online diabetes communities, including forums, social media groups, and support networks where people with diabetes can connect. These virtual platforms allow individuals to interact with others from around the world, providing a sense of connection and access to a wealth of shared knowledge.

- **Peer Mentoring Programs**: Some organizations offer peer mentoring programs where people with diabetes can be matched with a mentor who has experience managing the condition. This type of mentorship can provide emotional support, practical advice, and a sense of hope for individuals newly diagnosed with type 2 diabetes.

4. **Technology and Tools**

In today's digital age, technology can be a valuable part of building your support system. There are several tools and resources that can help individuals manage their diabetes more effectively.

- **Diabetes Management Apps**: Apps designed for diabetes management can help you track blood sugar levels, medications, meals, and physical activity. Many apps allow for data sharing with healthcare providers, making it easier to stay on top of your health and have meaningful discussions during appointments.

- **Telemedicine**: In cases where in-person visits may be challenging, telemedicine allows for remote consultations with healthcare providers. Virtual appointments make it easier to get timely advice, prescriptions, and follow-up care, without needing to travel to a clinic.

- **Online Tools for Meal Planning and Exercise**: Many online resources and apps can assist with meal planning, grocery shopping, and finding diabetes-friendly recipes. Additionally, fitness trackers and exercise apps can help monitor physical activity and encourage consistent exercise routines.

Conclusion

Managing type 2 diabetes is a lifelong journey, and building a strong support system is a crucial part of that journey. A support system that includes family, friends, healthcare professionals, support groups, and technology can provide the emotional, physical, and practical assistance needed to effectively manage the condition. It fosters a sense of community, reduces feelings of isolation, and helps individuals stay motivated and accountable.

By actively building and nurturing your support system, you create an environment where diabetes care becomes more manageable, sustainable, and even enjoyable. The encouragement and knowledge gained from a supportive network can improve not only diabetes outcomes but also overall well-being, providing the necessary tools to live a healthy, fulfilling life with type 2 diabetes.

Chapter 10: Living Your Best Life with Type 2 Diabetes

A diagnosis of type 2 diabetes (T2D) can be overwhelming, but it is by no means the end of a full and vibrant life. In fact, with proper management and a positive outlook, people with type 2 diabetes can live their best lives, thriving physically, mentally, and emotionally. Diabetes management involves not only controlling blood sugar levels but also embracing a holistic approach to health that includes lifestyle changes, emotional resilience, and a proactive attitude.

This article will explore how to live your best life with type 2 diabetes by focusing on practical tips for managing the condition, cultivating a healthy mindset, building strong support systems, and making lifestyle choices that promote overall well-being.

1. **Understanding Type 2 Diabetes**

Type 2 diabetes is a chronic condition in which the body either doesn't produce enough insulin or becomes resistant to it, leading to elevated blood sugar levels. Over time, high blood sugar can cause a range of health complications, such as heart disease, kidney damage, nerve problems, and vision impairment. However, it is possible to effectively manage the condition and prevent or delay complications through lifestyle adjustments, medication, and regular monitoring.

2. **Prioritizing Blood Sugar Management**

Blood sugar control is at the core of managing type 2 diabetes. By staying vigilant about blood glucose levels, individuals can prevent fluctuations that lead to long-term complications. Proper management often involves the following strategies:

a. **Monitoring Blood Glucose**

Regularly checking blood sugar levels is crucial to understanding how different foods, activities, medications, and stress affect your body. Home blood glucose monitoring is a simple and effective way to track how well your blood sugar levels are staying within the recommended range. Depending on the severity of your diabetes, your healthcare provider may advise you to check your blood sugar multiple times a day or a few times a week.

b. **Diet and Nutrition**

Eating a balanced, nutrient-dense diet is one of the most powerful ways to manage type 2 diabetes. Focusing on whole foods, including vegetables, fruits, whole grains, lean proteins, and healthy fats, can help stabilize blood sugar levels.

Carbohydrate counting, understanding the glycemic index of foods, and eating consistent meals throughout the day also play important roles in keeping blood sugar levels stable.

Key dietary tips for people with type 2 diabetes include:

- **Focus on fiber**: Fiber-rich foods, such as whole grains, legumes, and vegetables, help regulate blood sugar by slowing the absorption of sugar into the bloodstream.

- **Watch portion sizes**: Eating smaller portions can prevent blood sugar spikes after meals.

- **Limit processed sugars and carbs**: Processed sugars and refined carbohydrates can cause rapid increases in blood sugar levels. Choose whole foods that have a low glycemic index for better blood sugar control.

c. **Exercise and Physical Activity**

Physical activity is one of the most effective ways to manage blood sugar levels. Exercise increases insulin sensitivity, which means your body needs less insulin to manage blood sugar. It also helps with weight management, reduces inflammation, and improves cardiovascular health—important considerations for people with diabetes.

Aim for at least 150 minutes of moderate-intensity exercise per week, such as brisk walking, swimming, or cycling. Additionally, strength training exercises a couple of times a week can help build muscle mass, which further improves insulin sensitivity. It's important to find activities that you enjoy, so you're more likely to stick to an exercise routine.

d. **Medication and Treatment Plans**

Some individuals with type 2 diabetes may require medications to help manage blood sugar levels. These medications can include:

- **Metformin**: A common first-line medication that helps lower blood sugar by improving insulin sensitivity.

- **Sulfonylureas**: These medications stimulate the pancreas to release more insulin.

- **SGLT2 inhibitors**: Medications that help the kidneys remove excess sugar from the body through urine.

- **GLP-1 receptor agonists**: These drugs increase insulin production and reduce the amount of sugar produced by the liver.

If prescribed medication, it's essential to follow your doctor's recommendations and take the medications as directed. Your healthcare provider may adjust the treatment plan as needed to optimize blood sugar control.

3. **Mental and Emotional Well-being**

Managing type 2 diabetes is not only about physical health; mental and emotional well-being are equally important. The emotional challenges that come with managing a chronic illness can be significant, but there are ways to build resilience and develop a positive outlook.

a. **Managing Stress**

Stress can have a profound impact on blood sugar levels, often causing them to rise. Learning to manage stress effectively can help improve both mental and physical health. Techniques such as mindfulness, meditation, yoga, deep breathing exercises, and progressive muscle relaxation can help reduce stress and improve emotional well-being.

b. **Developing a Positive Mindset**

Having a positive attitude is essential for living your best life with diabetes. A positive mindset can help you approach the challenges of diabetes management with resilience and determination. Rather than viewing diabetes as a burden, try to embrace it as an opportunity to take charge of your health. Focus on the progress you've made and the things you can control, such as diet and exercise, instead of feeling overwhelmed by the things outside your control.

c. **Seeking Professional Support**

Mental health is a vital aspect of diabetes care. Many people with diabetes experience feelings of frustration, anxiety, or depression, which can negatively impact their ability to manage the condition effectively. If you're feeling overwhelmed, it's important to seek professional help. A therapist or counselor can help you cope with the emotional challenges of diabetes, and support groups provide an opportunity to connect with others who understand your experiences.

d. **Creating a Routine**

Having a structured daily routine helps manage the demands of diabetes. It can include regular meal times, exercise schedules, and consistent blood sugar monitoring. A predictable routine can reduce stress and increase adherence to diabetes management practices.

4. **Building a Strong Support System**

A strong support system is critical in managing type 2 diabetes. Building a network of people who understand your condition and can offer support is essential for emotional well-being and adherence to treatment plans.

a. **Family and Friends**

Sharing your diabetes journey with family and friends can foster understanding and encourage support. Educating loved ones about your condition and involving them in your care can make a significant difference. For example, they may help you prepare healthy meals, accompany you to medical appointments, or simply provide encouragement when you need it most.

b. **Healthcare Team**

Your healthcare providers, including doctors, diabetes educators, dietitians, and specialists, are integral members of your support system. They help guide your treatment plan, provide advice on managing blood sugar, and offer encouragement during difficult times. Regular check-ups and open communication with your healthcare team can help you stay on track with your diabetes management.

c. **Support Groups**

Diabetes support groups, whether in-person or online, offer a space for individuals to share their experiences, offer advice, and provide emotional support. Connecting with others who are navigating similar challenges can be incredibly empowering. Support groups can provide practical tips, a sense of community, and a platform for discussing concerns or celebrating successes.

5. **Living a Full Life Beyond Diabetes**

While managing type 2 diabetes is a significant part of daily life, it's important to remember that diabetes does not define you. You can continue to pursue your passions, engage in hobbies, and enjoy life to the fullest. Here are some ways to live your best life while managing diabetes:

a. **Pursuing Hobbies and Interests**

Engaging in activities that bring you joy is an important aspect of well-being. Whether it's painting, hiking, reading, or volunteering, taking time for yourself to enjoy hobbies helps reduce stress and enhances quality of life.

b. **Socializing and Staying Connected**

Socializing with friends and family helps combat feelings of isolation and loneliness. Engaging in social activities can also provide opportunities for physical activity, such as walking with a friend or participating in group fitness classes.

c. **Traveling and Exploring**

Having diabetes doesn't mean you can't travel or explore new places. With a little preparation, managing your diabetes while traveling is entirely possible. Make sure to carry all your medications, check blood sugar levels regularly, and plan your meals ahead of time. Many people with diabetes travel successfully by staying mindful of their health needs and prioritizing self-care.

6. **Conclusion**

Living your best life with type 2 diabetes requires a proactive approach to physical, emotional, and mental well-being. By focusing on blood sugar management, developing a positive mindset, building a strong support system, and embracing lifestyle changes, you can lead a fulfilling and vibrant life. Diabetes may be a part of your journey, but it doesn't have to define it. With the right mindset, support, and strategies, you can live your best life, achieving both health and happiness.

This comprehensive guide will empower you with knowledge, tools, and strategies to manage type 2 diabetes effectively. Each chapter is designed to provide actionable insights and encourage a proactive approach to health and wellness.